Hippocra

Aphorisms

Hippocrates

Translated by Francis Adams

Aphorisms

Section I

Life is short, and Art long; the crisis fleeting; experience perilous, and decision difficult. The physician must not only be prepared to do what is right himself, but also to make the patient, the attendants, and externals cooperate.

2. In disorders of the bowels and vomitings, occurring spontaneously, if the matters purged be such as ought to be purged, they do good, and are well borne; but if not, the contrary. And so artificial evacuations, if they consist of such matters as should be evacuated, do good, and are well borne; but if not, the contrary. One, then, ought to look to the country, the season, the age, and the diseases in which they are proper or not.

3. In the athletae, embonpoint, if carried to its utmost limit, is dangerous, for they cannot remain in the same state nor be stationary; and since, then, they can neither remain stationary nor improve, it only remains for them to get worse; for these reasons the embonpoint should be reduced without delay, that the body may again have a commencement of reparation. Neither should the evacuations, in their case, be carried to an extreme, for this also is dangerous, but only to such a point as the person's constitution can endure. In like manner, medicinal evacuations, if carried to an extreme, are dangerous; and again, a restorative course, if in the extreme, is dangerous.

4. A slender restricted diet is always dangerous in chronic diseases, and also in acute diseases, where it is not requisite. And again, a diet brought to the extreme point of attenuation is dangerous; and repletion, when in the extreme, is also dangerous.

5. In a restricted diet, patients who transgress are thereby more hurt (than in any other?); for every such transgression, whatever it may be, is followed by greater consequences than in a diet somewhat more generous. On this account, a very slender, regulated, and restricted diet is dangerous to persons in health, because they bear transgressions of it more difficultly. For this reason, a slender and restricted diet is generally more dangerous than one a little more liberal.

6. For extreme diseases, extreme methods of cure, as to restriction, are most suitable.

7. When the disease is very acute, it is attended with extremely severe symptoms in its first stage; and therefore an extremely attenuating diet must be used. When this is not the case, but it is allowable to give a more generous diet, we may depart as far from the severity of regimen as the disease, by its mildness, is removed from the extreme.

8. When the disease is at its height, it will then be necessary to use the most slender diet.

9. We must form a particular judgment of the patient, whether he will support the diet until the acme of the disease, and whether he will sink previously and not support the diet, or the disease will give way previously, and become less acute.

10. In those cases, then, which attain their acme speedily, a restricted diet should be enjoined at first; but in those cases which reach their acme later, we must retrench

3

at that period or a little before it; but previously we must allow a more generous diet to support the patient.

11. We must retrench during paroxysms, for to exhibit food would be injurious. And in all diseases having periodical paroxysms, we must restrict during the paroxysms.

12. The exacerbations and remissions will be indicated by the diseases, the seasons of the year, the reciprocation of the periods, whether they occur every day, every alternate day, or after a longer period, and by the supervening symptoms; as, for example, in pleuritic cases, expectoration, if it occur at the commencement, shortens the attack, but if it appear later, it prolongs the same; and in the same manner the urine, and alvine discharges, and sweats, according as they appear along with favorable or unfavorable symptoms, indicate diseases of a short or long duration.

13. Old persons endure fasting most easily; next, adults; young persons not nearly so well; and most especially infants, and of them such as are of a particularly lively spirit.

14. Growing bodies have the most innate heat; they therefore require the most food, for otherwise their bodies are wasted. In old persons the heat is feeble, and therefore they require little fuel, as it were, to the flame, for it would be extinguished by much. On this account, also, fevers in old persons are not equally acute, because their bodies are cold.

15. In winter and spring the bowels are naturally the hottest, and the sleep most prolonged; at these seasons, then, the most sustenance is to be administered; for as the belly has then most innate heat, it stands in need of most food. The well-known facts with regard to young persons and the athletae prove this.

16. A humid regimen is befitting in all febrile diseases, and particularly in children, and others accustomed to live on such a diet.

17. We must consider, also, in which cases food is to be given once or twice a day, and in greater or smaller quantities, and at intervals. Something must be conceded to habit, to season, to country, and to age.

18. Invalids bear food worst during summer and autumn, most easily in winter, and next in spring.

19. Neither give nor enjoin anything to persons during periodical paroxysms, but abstract from the accustomed allowance before the crisis.

20. When things are at the crisis, or when they have just passed it, neither move the bowels, nor make any innovation in the treatment, either as regards purgatives or any other such stimulants, but let things alone.

21. Those things which require to be evacuated should be evacuated, wherever they most tend, by the proper outlets.

22. We must purge and move such humors as are concocted, not such as are unconcocted, unless they are struggling to get out, which is mostly not the case.

23. The evacuations are to be judged of not by their quantity, but whether they be such as they should be, and how they are borne. And when proper to carry the evacuation to deliquium animi, this also should be done, provided the patient can support it.

24. Use purgative medicines sparingly in acute diseases, and at the commencement, and not without proper circumspection.

25. If the matters which are purged be such as should be purged, the evacuation is beneficial, and easily borne; but, not withstanding, if otherwise, with difficulty.

SECTION II.

1. In whatever disease sleep is laborious, it is a deadly symptom; but if sleep does good, it is not deadly.

2. When sleep puts an end to delirium, it is a good symptom.

3. Both sleep and insomnolency, when immoderate, are bad.

4. Neither repletion, nor fasting, nor anything else, is good when more than natural.

5. Spontaneous lassitude indicates disease.

6. Persons who have a painful affection in any part of the body, and are in a great measure sensible of the pain, are disordered in intellect.

7. Those bodies which have been slowly emaciated should be slowly recruited; and those which have been quickly emaciated should be quickly recruited.

8. When a person after a disease takes food, but does not improve in strength, it indicates that the body uses more food than is proper; but if this happen when he does not take food, it is to be understood evacuation is required.

9. When one wishes to purge, he should put the body into a fluent state.

10. Bodies not properly cleansed, the more you nourish the more you injure.

11. It is easier to fill up with drink than with food.

12. What remains in diseases after the crisis is apt to produce relapses.

13. Persons in whom a crisis takes place pass the night preceding the paroxysm uncomfortably, but the succeeding night generally more comfortably.

14. In fluxes of the bowels, a change of the dejections does good, unless the change be of a bad character.

15. When the throat is diseased, or tubercles (phymata) form on the body, attention must paid to the secretions; for if they be bilious, the disease affects the general system; but if they resemble those of a healthy person, it is safe to give nourishing food.

16. When in a state of hunger, one ought not to undertake labor.

17. When more food than is proper has been taken, it occasions disease; this is shown by the treatment.

18. From food which proves nourishing to the body either immediately or shortly, the dejections also are immediate.

19. In acute diseases it is not quite safe to prognosticate either death or recovery.

20. Those who have watery discharges from their bowels when young have dry when they are old; and those who have dry discharges when they are young will have watery when they are old.

21. Drinking strong wine cures hunger.

22. Diseases which arise from repletion are cured by depletion; and those that arise from depletion are cured by repletion; and in general, diseases are cured by their contraries.

23. Acute disease come to a crisis in fourteen days.

24. The fourth day is indicative of the seventh; the eighth is the commencement of the second week; and hence, the eleventh being the fourth of the second week, is also indicative; and again, the seventeenth is indicative, as being the fourth from the fourteenth, and the seventh from the eleventh.

25. The summer quartans are, for the most part, of short duration; but the autumnal are protracted, especially those occurring near the approach of winter.

26. It is better that a fever succeed to a convulsion, than a convulsion to a fever.

27. We should not trust ameliorations in diseases when they are not regular, nor be much afraid of bad symptoms which occur in an irregular form; for such are commonly inconstant, and do not usually continue, nor have any duration.

28. In fevers which are not altogether slight, it is a bad symptom for the body to remain without any diminution of bulk, or to be wasted beyond measure; for the one state indicates a protracted disease, and the other weakness of body.

29. If it appear that evacuations are required, they should be made at the commencement of diseases; at the acme it is better to be quiet.

30. Toward the commencement and end of diseases all the symptoms are weaker, and toward the acme they are stronger.

31. When a person who is recovering from a disease has a good appetite, but his body does not improve in condition, it is a bad symptom.

32. For the most part, all persons in ill health, who have a good appetite at the commencement, but do not improve, have a bad appetite again toward the end; whereas, those who have a very bad appetite at the commencement, and afterward acquire a good appetite, get better off.

33. In every disease it is a good sign when the patient's intellect is sound, and he is disposed to take whatever food is offered to him; but the contrary is bad.

34. In diseases, there is less danger when the disease is one to which the patient's constitution, habit, age, and the season are allied, than when it is one to which they are not allied.

35. In all diseases it is better that the umbilical and hypogastric regions preserve their fullness; and it is a bad sign when they are very slender and emaciated; in the latter case it is dangerous to administer purgatives.

36. Persons in good health quickly lose their strength by taking purgative medicines, or using bad food.

37. Purgative medicines agree ill with persons in good health.

38. An article of food or drink which is slightly worse, but more palatable, is to be preferred to such as are better but less palatable.

39. Old have fewer complaints than young; but those chronic diseases which do befall them generally never leave them.

40. Catarrhs and coryza in very old people are not concocted.

41. Persons who have had frequent and severe attacks of swooning, without any manifest cause, die suddenly.

42. It is impossible to remove a strong attack of apoplexy, and not easy to remove a weak attack.

43. Of persons who have been suspended by the neck, and are in a state of insensibility, but not quite dead, those do not recover who have foam at the mouth.

44. Persons who are naturally very fat are apt to die earlier than those who are slender.

45. Epilepsy in young persons is most frequently removed by changes of air, of country, and of modes of life.

46. Of two pains occurring together, not in the same part of the body, the stronger weakens the other.

47. Pains and fevers occur rather at the formation of pus than when it is already formed.

48. In every movement of the body, whenever one begins to endure pain, it will be relieved by rest.

49. Those who are accustomed to endure habitual labors, although they be weak or old, bear them better than strong and young persons who have not been so accustomed.

50. Those things which one has been accustomed to for a long time, although worse than things which one is not accustomed to, usually give less disturbance; but a change must sometimes be made to things one is not accustomed to.

51. To evacuate, fill up, heat, cool, or otherwise, move the body in any way much and suddenly, is dangerous; and whatever is excessive is inimical to nature; but whatever is done by little and little is safe, more especially when a transition is made from one thing to another.

52. When doing everything according to indications, although things may not turn out agreeably to indication, we should not change to another while the original appearances remain.

53. Those persons who have watery discharges from the bowels when they are young, come off better than those who have dry; but in old age they come off worse, for the bowels in aged persons are usually dried up.

54. Largeness of person in youth is noble and not unbecoming; but in old age it is inconvenient, and worse than a smaller structure.

SECTION III.

1. The changes of the season mostly engender diseases, and in the seasons great changes either of heat or of cold, and the rest agreeably to the same rule.

2. Of natures (temperaments?), some are well — or ill-adapted for summer, and some for winter.

3. Of diseases and ages, certain of them are well — or ill-adapted to different seasons, places, and kinds of diet.

7

4. In the seasons, when during the same day there is at one time heat and at another time cold, the diseases of autumn may be expected.

5. South winds induce dullness of hearing, dimness of visions, heaviness of the head, torpor, and languor; when these prevail, such symptoms occur in diseases. But if the north wind prevail, coughs, affections of the throat, hardness of the bowels, dysuria attended with rigors, and pains of the sides and breast occur. When this wind prevails, all such symptoms may be expected in diseases.

6. When summer is like spring, much sweating may be expected in fevers.

7. Acute diseases occur in droughts; and if the summer be particularly such, according to the constitution which it has given to the year, for the most part such diseases maybe expected.

8. In seasons which are regular, and furnish the productions of the season at the seasonable time, the diseases are regular, and come readily to a crisis; but in inconstant seasons, the diseases are irregular, and come to a crisis with difficulty.

9. In autumn, diseases are most acute, and most mortal, on the whole. The spring is most healthy, and least mortal.

10. Autumn is a bad season for persons in consumption.

11. With regard to the seasons, if the winter be of a dry and northerly character, and the spring rainy and southerly, in summer there will necessarily be acute fevers, ophthalmies, and dysenteries, especially in women, and in men of a humid temperament.

12. If the but the spring dry and northerly, women whose term of delivery should be in spring, have abortions from any slight cause; and those who reach their full time, bring forth children who are feeble, and diseased, so that they either die presently, or, if they live, are puny and unhealthy. Other people are subject to dysenteries and ophthalmies, and old men to catarrhs, which quickly cut them off.

13. If the summer be dry and northerly and the autumn rainy and southerly, headaches occur in winter, with coughs, hoarsenesses, coryzae, and in some cases consumptions.

14. But if the autumn be northerly and dry, it agrees well with persons of a humid temperament, and with women; but others will be subject to dry ophthalmies, acute fevers, coryzae, and in some cases melancholy.

15. Of the constitutions of the year, the dry, upon the whole, are more healthy than the rainy, and attended with less mortality.

16. The diseases which occur most frequently in rainy seasons are, protracted fevers, fluxes of the bowels, mortifications, epilepsies, apoplexies, and quinsies; and in dry, consumptive diseases, ophthalmies, arthritic diseases, stranguries, and dysenteries.

17. With regard to the states of the weather which continue but for a day, that which is northerly, braces the body, giving it tone, agility, and color, improves the sense of hearing, dries up the bowels, pinches the eyes, and aggravates any previous pain which may have been seated in the chest. But the southerly relaxes the body, and renders it humid, brings on dullness of hearing, heaviness of the head, and vertigo,

impairs the movements of the eyes and the whole body, and renders the alvine discharges watery.

18. With regard to the seasons, in spring and in the commencement of summer, children and those next to them in age are most comfortable, and enjoy best health; in summer and during a certain portion of autumn, old people; during the remainder of the autumn and in winter, those of the intermediate ages.

19. All diseases occur at all seasons of the year, but certain of them are more apt to occur and be exacerbated at certain seasons.

20. The diseases of spring are, maniacal, melancholic, and epileptic disorders, bloody flux, quinsy, coryza, hoarseness, cough, leprosy, lichen alphos, exanthemata mostly ending in ulcerations, tubercles, and arthritic diseases.

21. Of summer, certain of these, and continued, ardent, and tertian fevers, most especially vomiting, diarrhoea, ophthalmy, pains of the ears, ulcerations of the mouth, mortifications of the privy parts, and the sudamina.

22. Of autumn, most of the summer, quartan, and irregular fevers, enlarged spleen, dropsy, phthisis, strangury, lientery, dysentery, sciatica, quinsy, asthma, ileus, epilepsy, maniacal and melancholic disorders.

23. Of winter, pleurisy, pneumonia, coryza, hoarseness, cough, pains of the chest, pains of the ribs and loins, headache, vertigo, and apoplexy.

24. In the different ages the following complaints occur: to little and new-born children, aphthae, vomiting, coughs, sleeplessness, frights inflammation of the navel, watery discharges from the ears.

25. At the approach of dentition, pruritus of the gums, fevers, convulsions, diarrhoea, especially when cutting the canine teeth, and in those who are particularly fat, and have constipated bowels.

26. To persons somewhat older, affections of the tonsils, incurvation of the spine at the vertebra next the occiput, asthma, calculus, round worms, ascarides, acrochordon, satyriasmus, struma, and other tubercles (phymata), but especially the aforesaid.

27. To persons of a more advanced age, and now on the verge of manhood, the most of these diseases, and, moreover, more chronic fevers, and epistaxis.

28. Young people for the most part have a crisis in their complaints, some in forty days, some in seven months, some in seven years, some at the approach to puberty; and such complaints of children as remain, and do not pass away about puberty, or in females about the commencement of menstruation, usually become chronic.

29. To persons past boyhood, haemoptysis, phthisis, acute fevers, epilepsy, and other diseases, but especially the aforementioned.

30. To persons beyond that age, asthma, pleurisy, pneumonia, lethargy, phrenitis, ardent fevers, chronic diarrhoea, cholera, dysentery, lientery, hemorrhoids.

31. To old people dyspnoea, catarrhs accompanied with coughs, dysuria, pains of the joints, nephritis, vertigo, apoplexy, cachexia, pruritus of the whole body, insomnolency, defluxions of the bowels, of the eyes, and of the nose, dimness of sight, cataract (glaucoma), and dullness of hearing.

9

1. We must purge pregnant women, if matters be turgid (in a state of orgasm?), from the fourth to the seventh month, but less freely in the latter; in the first and last stages of pregnancy it should be avoided.

2. In purging we should bring away such matters from the body as it would be advantageous had they come away spontaneously; but those of an opposite character should be stopped.

3. If the matters which are purged be such as should be purged, it is beneficial and well borne; but if the contrary, with difficulty.

4. We should rather purge upward in summer, and downward in winter.

5. About the time of the dog-days, and before it, the administration of purgatives is unsuitable.

6. Lean persons who are easily made to vomit should be purged upward, avoiding the winter season.

7. Persons who are difficult to vomit, and are moderately fat, should be purged downward, avoiding the summer season.

8. We must be guarded in purging phthisical persons upward.

9. And from the same mode of reasoning, applying the opposite rule to melancholic persons, we must purge them freely downward.

10. In very acute diseases, if matters be in a state of orgasm, we may purge on the first day, for it is a bad thing to procrastinate in such cases.

11. Those cases in which there are tormina, pains about the umbilicus, and pains about the loins, not removed either by purgative medicines or otherwise, usually terminate in dry dropsy.

12. It is a bad thing to purge upward in winter persons whose bowels are in a state of lientery.

13. Persons who are not easily purged upward by the hellebores, should have their bodies moistened by plenty of food and rest before taking the draught.

14. When one takes a draught of hellebore, one should be made to move more about, and indulge less in sleep and repose. Sailing on the sea shows that motion disorders the body.

15. When you wish the hellebore to act more, move the body, and when to stop, let the patient get sleep and rest.

16. Hellebore is dangerous to persons whose flesh is sound, for it induces convulsion.

17. Anorexia, heartburn, vertigo, and a bitter taste of the mouth, in a person free from fever, indicate the want of purging upward.

18. Pains seated above the diaphragm indicate purging upward, and those below it, downward.

19. Persons who have no thirst while under the action of a purgative medicine, do not cease from being purged until they become thirsty.

20. If persons free from fever be seized with tormina, heaviness of the knees, and pains of the loins, this indicates that purging downward is required.

21. Alvine dejections which are black, like blood, taking place spontaneously, either with or without fever, are very bad; and the more numerous and unfavorable the colors, so much the worse; when with medicine it is better, and a variety of colors in this case is not bad.

22. When black bile is evacuated in the beginning of any disease whatever, either upward or downward, it is a mortal symptom.

23. In persons attenuated from any disease, whether acute or chronic, or from wounds, or any other cause, if there be a discharge either of black bile, or resembling black blood, they die on the following day.

24. Dysentery, if it commence with black bile, is mortal.

25. Blood discharged upward, whatever be its character, is a bad symptom, but downward it is (more?) favorable, and so also black dejections.

26. If in a person ill of dysentery, substances resembling flesh be discharged from the bowels, it is a mortal symptom.

27. In whatever cases of fever there is a copious hemorrhage from whatever channel, the bowels are in a loose state during convalescence.

28. In all cases whatever, bilious discharges cease if deafness supervenes, and in all cases deafness ceases when bilious discharges supervene.

29. Rigors which occur on the sixth day have a difficult crisis.

30. Diseases attended with paroxysms, if at the same hour that the fever leaves it return again next day, are of difficult crisis.

31. In febrile diseases attended with a sense of lassitude, deposits form about the joints, and especially those of the jaws.

32. In convalescents from diseases, if any part be pained, there deposits are formed.

33. But if any part be in a painful state previous to the illness, there the disease fixes.

34. If a person laboring under a fever, without any swelling in the fauces, be seized with a sense of suffocation suddenly, it is a mortal symptom.

35. If in a person with fever, the become suddenly distorted, and he cannot swallow unless with difficulty, although no swelling be present, it is a mortal symptom.

36. Sweats, in febrile diseases, are favorable, if they set in on the third, fifth, seventh, ninth, eleventh, fourteenth, seventeenth, twenty-first, twenty-seventh, and thirty-fourth day, for these sweats prove a crisis to the disease; but sweats not occurring thus, indicate pain, a protracted disease, and relapses.

37. Cold sweats occurring with an acute fever, indicate death; and along with a milder one, a protracted disease.

38. And in whatever part of the body there is a sweat, it shows that the disease is seated there.

39. And in whatever part of the body heat or cold is seated, there is disease.

40. And wherever there are changes in the whole body, and if the body be alternately cold and hot, or if one color succeed another, this indicates a protracted disease.

41. A copious sweat after sleep occuring without any manifest cause, indicates that the body is using too much food. But if it occur when one is not taking food, it indicates that evacuation is required.

42. A copious sweat, whether hot or cold, flowing continuously, indicates, the cold a greater, and the hot a lesser disease.

43. Fevers, not of the intermittent type, which are exacerbated on the third day, are dangerous; but if they intermit in any form, this indicates that they are not dangerous.

44. In cases attended with protracted fevers, tubercles (phymata) or pains occur about the joints.

45. When tubercles (phymata) or pains attack the joints after fevers, such persons are using too much food.

46. If in a fever not of the intermittent type a rigor seize a person already much debilitated, it is mortal.

47. In fevers not of the intermittent type, expectorations which are livid bloody, fetid and bilious, are all bad; but if evacuated properly, they are favorable. So it is with the alvine evacuations and the urine. But if none of the proper excretions take place by these channels, it is bad.

48. In fevers not of the intermittent type, if the external parts be cold, but the internal be burnt up, and if there be thirst, it is a mortal symptom.

49. In a fever not of the intermittent type, if a lip, an eye-brow, an eye, or the nose, be distorted; or if there be loss of sight or of hearing, and the patient be in a weak state- whatever of these symptoms occur, death is at hand.

50. Apostemes in fevers which are not resolved at the first crisis, indicate a protracted disease.

51. When in a fever not of the intermittent type dyspnoea and delirium come on, the case is mortal.

52. When persons in fevers, or in other illnesses, shed tears voluntarily, it is nothing out of place; but when they shed tears involuntarily, it is more so.

53. In whatever cases of fever very viscid concretions form about the teeth, the fevers turn out to be particularly strong.

54. In whatever case of ardent fever dry coughs of a tickling nature with slight expectoration are long protracted, there is usually not much thirst.

55. All fevers complicated with buboes are bad, except ephemerals.

56. Sweat supervening in a case of the fever ceasing, is bad, for the disease is protracted, and it indicates more copious humors.

57. Fever supervening in a case of confirmed spasm, or of tetanus, removes the disease.

58. A rigor supervening in a case of ardent fever, produces resolution of it.

59. A true tertian comes to a crisis in seven periods at furthest.

60. When in fevers there is deafness, if blood run from the nostrils, or the bowels become disordered, it carries off the disease.

61. In a febrile complaint, if the fever do not leave on the odd days, it relapses.

62. When jaundice supervenes in fevers before the seventh day, it a bad symptom, unless there be watery discharges from the bowels.

63. In whatever cases of fever rigors occur during the day, the fevers come to a resolution during the day.

64. When in cases of fever jaundice occurs on the seventh, the ninth, the eleventh, or the fourteenth day, it is a good symptom, provided the hypochondriac region be not hard. Otherwise it is not a good symptom.

65. A strong heat about the stomach and cardialgia are bad symptoms in fevers.

66. In acute fevers, spasms, and strong pains about the bowels are bad symptoms.

67. In fevers, frights after sleep, or convulsions, are a bad symptom.

68. In fevers, a stoppage of the respiration is a bad symptom, for it indicates convulsions.

69. When the urine is thick, grumoss, and scanty in cases not free from fever a copious discharge of thinner urine proves beneficial. Such a discharge more commonly takes place when the urine has had a sediment from the first, or soon after the commencement.

70. When in fevers the urine is turbid, like that of a beast of burden, in such a case there either is or will be headache.

71. In cases which come to a crisis on the seventh day, the urine has a red nubecula on the fourth day, and the other symptoms accordingly.

72. When the urine is transparent and white, it is bad; it appears principally in cases of phrenitis.

73. When the hypochondriac region is affected with meteorism and borborygmi, should pain of the loins supervene, the bowels get into a loose and watery state, unless there be an eruption of flatus or a copious evacuation of urine. These things occur in fevers.

74. When there is reason to expect that an abscess will form in joints, the abscess is carried off by a copious discharge of urine, which is thick, and becomes white, like what begins to form in certain cases of quartan fever, attended with a sense of lassitude. It is also speedily carried off by a hemorrhage from the nose.

75. Blood or pus in the urine indicates ulceration either of the kidneys or of the bladder.

76. When small fleshy substances like hairs are discharged along with thick urine, these substances come from the kidneys.

77. In those cases where there are furfuraceous particles discharged along with thick urine, there is scabies of the bladder.

78. In those cases where there is a spontaneous discharge of bloody urine, it indicates rupture of a small vein in the kidneys.

79. In those cases where there is a sandy sediment in the urine, there is calculus in the bladder (or kidneys).

80. If a patient pass blood and clots in his urine, and have strangury, and if a pain seize the hypogastric region and perineum, the parts about the bladder are affected.

81. If a patient pass blood, pus, and scales, in the urine, and if it have a heavy smell, ulceration of the bladder is indicated.

82. When tubercles form in the urethra, if these suppurate and burst, there is relief.

83. When much urine is passed during the night, it indicates that the alvine evacuations are scanty.

SECTION V.

1. A spasm from taking hellebore is of a fatal nature.

2. Spasm supervening on a wound is fatal.

3. A convulsion, or hiccup, supervening on a copious discharge of blood is bad.

4. A convulsion, or hiccup, supervening upon hypercatharsis is bad.

5. If a drunken person suddenly lose his speech, he will die convulsed, unless fever come on, or he recover his speech at the time when the consequences of a debauch pass off.

6. Such persons as are seized with tetanus die within four days, or if they pass these they recover.

7. Those cases of epilepsy which come on before puberty may undergo a change; but those which come on after twenty-five years of age, for the most part terminate in death.

8. In pleuritic affections, when the disease is not purged off in fourteen days, it usually terminates in empyema.

9. Phthisis most commonly occurs between the ages of eighteen and thirty-five years.

10. Persons who escape an attack of quinsy, and when the disease is turned upon the lungs, die in seven days; or if they pass these they become affected with empyema.

11. In persons affected with phthisis, if the sputa which they cough up have a heavy smell when poured upon coals, and if the hairs of the head fall off, the case will prove fatal.

12. Phthisical persons, the hairs of whose head fall off, die if diarrhoea set in.

13. In persons who cough up frothy blood, the discharge of it comes from the lungs.

14. Diarrhoea attacking a person affected with phthisis is a mortal symptom.

15. Persons who become affected with empyema after pleurisy, if they get clear of it in forty days from the breaking of it, escape the disease; but if not, it passes into phthisis.

16. Heat produces the following bad effects on those who use it frequently: enervation of the fleshy parts, impotence of the nerves, torpor of the understanding, hemorrhages, deliquia, and, along with these, death.

17. Cold induces convulsions, tetanus, mortification, and febrile rigors.

14

18. Cold is inimical to the bones, the teeth, the nerves, the brain, and the spinal marrow, but heat is beneficial.

19. Such parts as have been congealed should be heated, except where there either is a hemorrhage, or one is expected.

20. Cold pinches ulcers, hardens the skin, occasions pain which does not end in suppuration, blackens, produces febrile rigors, convulsions, and tetanus.

21. In the case of a muscular youth having tetanus without a wound, during the midst of summer, it sometimes happens that the allusion of a large quantity of cold water recalls the heat. Heat relieves these diseases.

22. Heat is suppurative, but not in all kinds of sores, but when it is, it furnishes the greatest test of their being free from danger. It softens the skin, makes it thin, removes pain, soothes rigor, convulsions, and tetanus. It removes affections of the head, and heaviness of it. It is particularly efficacious in fractures of the bones, especially of those which have been exposed, and most especially in wounds of the head, and in mortifications and ulcers from cold; in herpes exedens, of the anus, the privy parts, the womb, the bladder, in all these cases heat is agreeable, and brings matters to a crisis; but cold is prejudicial, and does mischief.

23. Cold water is to be applied in the following cases; when there is a hemorrhage, or when it is expected, but not applied to the spot, but around the spot whence the blood flows; and in inflammations and inflammatory affections, inclining to a red and subsaguineous color, and consisting of fresh blood, in these cases it is to be applied but it occasions mortification in old cases; and in erysipelas not attended with ulceration, as it proves injurious to erysipelas when ulcerated.

24. Cold things, such as snow and ice, are inimical to the chest, being provocative of coughs, of discharges of blood, and of catarrhs.

25. Swellings and pains in the joints, ulceration, those of a gouty nature, and sprains, are generally improved by a copious affusion of cold water, which reduces the swelling, and removes the pain; for a moderate degree of numbness removes pain.

26. The lightest water is that which is quickly heated and quickly cooled.

27. When persons have intense thirst, it is a good thing if they can sleep off the desire of drinking.

28. Fumigation with aromatics promotes menstruation, and would be useful in many other cases, if it did not occasion heaviness of the head.

29. Women in a state of pregnancy may be purged, if there be any urgent necessity (or, if the humors be in a state of orgasm?), from the fourth to the seventh month, but less so in the latter case. In the first and last periods it must be avoided.

30. It proves fatal to a woman in a state of pregnancy, if she be seized with any of the acute diseases.

31. If a woman with child be bled, she will have an abortion, and this will be the more likely to happen, the larger the foetus.

32. Haemoptysis in a woman is removed by an eruption of the menses.

33. In a woman when there is a stoppage the menses, a discharge of blood from the nose is good.

34. When a pregnant woman has a violent diarrhoea, there is danger of her miscarrying.

35. Sneezing occurring to a woman affected with hysterics, and in difficult labor, is a good symptom.

36. When the menstrual discharge is of a bad color and irregular, it indicates that the woman stands in need of purging.

37. In a pregnant woman, if the breasts suddenly lose their fullness, she has a miscarriage.

38. If, in a woman pregnant with twins, either of her breasts lose its fullness, she will part with one of her children; and if it be the right breast which becomes slender, it will be the male child, or if the left, the female.

39. If a woman who is not with child, nor has brought forth, have milk, her menses are obstructed.

40. In women, blood collected in the breasts indicates madness.

41. If you wish to ascertain if a woman be with child, give her hydromel to drink when she is going to sleep, and has not taken supper, and if she be seized with tormina in the belly, she is with child, but otherwise she is not pregnant.

42. A woman with child, if it be a male, has a good color, but if a female, she has a bad color.

43. If erysipelas of the womb seize a woman with child, it will probably prove fatal.

44. Women who are very lean, have miscarriages when they prove with child, until they get into better condition.

45. When women, in a moderate condition of body, miscarry in the second or third month, without any obvious cause, their cotyledones are filled with mucosity, and cannot support the weight of the foetus, but are broken asunder.

46. Such women as are immoderately fat, and do not prove with child, in them it is because the epiploon (fat?) blocks up the mouth of the womb, and until it be reduced, they do not conceive.

47. If the portion of the uterus seated near the hip-joint suppurate, it gets into a state requiring to be treated with tents.

48. The male foetus is usually seated in the right, and the female in the left side.

49. To procure the expulsion of the secundines, apply a sternutatory, and shut the nostrils and mouth.

50. If you wish to stop the menses in a woman, apply as large a cupping instrument as possible to the breasts.

51. When women are with child, the mouth of their womb is closed.

52. If in a woman with child, much milk flow from the breasts, it indicates that the foetus is weak; but if the breasts be firm, it indicates that the foetus is in a more healthy state.

53. In women that are about to miscarry, the breasts become slender; but if again they become hard, there will be pain, either in the breasts, or in the hip-joints, or in the eyes, or in the knees, and they will not miscarry.

54. When the mouth of the uterus is hard, it is also necessarily shut.

55. Women with child who are seized with fevers, and who are greatly emaciated, without any (other?) obvious cause, have difficult and dangerous labors, and if they miscarry, they are in danger.

56. In the female flux (immoderate menstruation?), if convulsion and deliquium come on, it is bad.

57. When the menses are excessive, diseases take place, and when the menses are stopped, diseases from the uterus take place.

58. Strangury supervenes upon inflammation of the rectum, and of the womb, and strangury supervenes upon suppuration of the kidney, and hiccup upon inflammation of the liver.

59. If a woman do not conceive, and wish to ascertain whether she can conceive, having wrapped her up in blankets, fumigate below, and if it appear that the scent passes through the body to the nostrils and mouth, know that of herself she is not unfruitful.

60. If woman with a child have her courses, it is impossible that the child can be healthy.

61. If a woman's courses be suppressed, and neither rigor nor fever has followed, but she has been affected with nausea, you may reckon her to be with child.

62. Women who have the uterus cold and dense (compact?) do not conceive; and those also who have the uterus humid, do not conceive, for the semen is extinguished, and in women whose uterus is very dry, and very hot, the semen is lost from the want of food; but women whose uterus is in an intermediate state between these temperaments prove fertile.

63. And in like manner with respect to males; for either, owing to the laxity of the body, the pneuma is dissipated outwardly, so as not to propel the semen, or, owing to its density, the fluid (semen?) does not pass outwardly; or, owing to coldness, it is not heated so as to collect in its proper place (seminal vessels?), or, owing to its heat, the very same thing happens.

64. It is a bad thing to give milk to persons having headache, and it is also bad to give it in fevers, and to persons whose hypochondria are swelled up, and troubled with borborygmi, and to thirsty persons; it is bad also, when given to those who have bilious discharges in acute fevers, and to those who have copious discharges of blood; but it is suitable in phthisical cases, when not attended with very much fever; it is also to be given in fevers of a chronic and weak nature, when none of the aforementioned symptoms are present, and the patients are excessively emaciated.

65. When swellings appear on wounds, such cases are not likely to be attacked either with convulsions, or delirium, but when these disappear suddenly, if situated behind, spasms and tetanus supervene, and if before, mania, acute pains of the sides, or suppurations, or dysentery, if the swellings be rather red.

66. When no swelling appears on severe and bad wounds, it is a great evil.

67. In such cases, the soft are favorable; and crude, unfavorable.

68. When a person is pained in the back part of the head, he is benefited by having the straight vein in the forehead opened.

69. Rigors commence in women, especially at the loins, and spread by the back to the head; and in men also, rather in the posterior than the anterior side of the body, as from the arms and thighs; the skin there is rare, as is obvious from the growth of hair on them.

70. Persons attacked with quartans are not readily attacked with convulsions, or if previously attacked with convulsions, they cease if a quartan supervene.

71. In those persons in whom the skin is stretched, and parched and hard, the disease terminates without sweats; but in those in whom the skin is loose and rare, it terminates with sweats.

72. Persons disposed to jaundice are not very subject to flatulence.

SECTION VI.

1. In cases of chronic lientery, acid eructations supervening when there were none previously, is a good symptom.

2. Persons whose noses are naturally watery, and their seed watery, have rather a deranged state of health; but those in the opposite state, a more favorable.

3. In protracted cases of dysentery, loathing of food is a bad symptom, and still worse, if along with fever.

4. Ulcers, attended with a falling off of the hair, are mali moris.

5. It deserves to be considered whether the pains in the sides, and in the breasts, and in the other parts, differ much from one another.

6. Diseases about the kidneys and bladder are cured with difficulty in old men.

7. Pains occurring about the stomach, the more superficial they are, the more slight are they; and the less superficial, the more severe.

8. In dropsical persons, ulcers forming on the body are not easily healed.

9. Broad exanthemata are not very itchy.

10. In a person having a painful spot in the head, with intense cephalalgia, pus or water running from the nose, or by the mouth, or at the ears, removes the disease.

11. Hemorrhoids appearing in melancholic and nephritic affections are favorable.

12. When a person has been cured of chronic hemorrhoids, unless one be left, there is danger of dropsy or phthisis supervening.

13. Sneezing coming on, in the case of a person afflicted with hiccup, removes the hiccup.

14. In a case of dropsy, when the water runs by the veins into the belly, it removes the disease.

15. In confirmed diarrhoea, vomiting, when it comes on spontaneously, removes the diarrhoea.

16. A diarrhoea supervening in a confirmed case of pleurisy or pneumonia is bad.

17. It is a good thing in ophthalmy for the patient to be seized with diarrhoea.

18. A severe wound of the bladder, of the brain, of the heart, of the diaphragm, of the small intestines, of the stomach, and of the liver, is deadly.

19. When a bone, cartilage, nerve, the slender part of the jaw, or prepuce, are cut out, the part is neither restored, nor does it unite.

20. If blood be poured out preternaturally into a cavity, it must necessarily become corrupted.

21. In maniacal affections, if varices or hemorrhoids come on, they remove the mania.

22. Those ruptures in the back which spread down to the elbows are removed by venesection.

23. If a fright or despondency lasts for a long time, it is a melancholic affection.

24. If any of the intestines be transfixed, it does not unite.

25. It is not a good sign for an erysipelas spreading outwardly to be determined inward; but for it to be determined outward from within is good.

26. In whatever cases of ardent fever tremors occur, they are carried off by a delirium.

27. Those cases of empyema or dropsy which are treated by incision or the cautery, if the water or pus flow rapidly all at once, certainly prove fatal.

28. Eunuchs do not take the gout, nor become bald.

29. A woman does not take the gout, unless her menses be stopped.

30. A young man does not take the gout until he indulges in coition.

31. Pains of the eyes are removed by drinking pure wine, or the bath, or a fomentation, or venesection, or purging.

32. Persons whose speech has become impaired are likely to be seized with chronic diarrhoea.

33. Persons having acid eructations are not very apt to be seized with pleurisy.

34. Persons who have become bald are not subject to large varices; but should varices supervene upon persons who are bald, their hair again grows thick.

35. Hiccup supervening in dropsical cases is bad.

36. Venesection cures dysuria; open the internal veins of the arm.

37. It is a good symptom when swelling on the outside of the neck seizes a person very ill of quinsy, for the disease is turned outwardly.

38. It is better not to apply any treatment in cases of occult cancer; for, if treated, the patients die quickly; but if not treated, they hold out for a long time.

39. Convulsions take place either from repletion or depletion; and so it is with hiccup.

40. When pains, without inflammation, occur about the hypochondria, in such cases, fever supervening removes the pain.

41. When pus formed anywhere in the body does not point, this is owing to the thickness of the part.

42. In cases of jaundice, it is a bad symptom when the liver becomes indurated.

43. When persons having large spleens are seized with dysentery, and if the dysentery pass into a chronic state, either dropsy or lientery supervenes, and they die.

44. When ileus comes on in a case of strangury, they prove fatal in seven days, unless, fever supervening, there be a copious discharge of urine.

45. When ulcers continue open for a year or upward, there must necessarily be exfoliation of bone, and the cicatrices are hollow.

46. Such persons as become hump-backed from asthma or cough before puberty, die.

47. Persons who are benefited by venesection or purging, should be bled or purged in spring.

48. In enlargement of the spleen, it is a good symptom when dysentery comes on.

49. In gouty affections, the inflammation subsides in the course of forty days.

50. When the brain is severely wounded, fever and vomiting of bile necessarily supervene.

51. When persons in good health are suddenly seized with pains in the head, and straightway are laid down speechless, and breathe with stertor, they die in seven days, unless fever come on.

52. We must attend to the appearances of the eyes in sleep, as presented from below; for if a portion of the white be seen between the closed eyelids, and if this be not connected with diarrhoea or severe purging, it is a very bad and mortal symptom.

53. Delirium attended with laughter is less dangerous than delirium attended with a serious mood.

54. In acute diseases, complicated with fever, a moaning respiration is bad.

55. For the most part, gouty affections rankle in spring and in autumn.

56. In melancholic affections, determinations of the humor which occasions them produce the following diseases; either apoplexy of the whole body, or convulsion, or madness, or blindness.

57. Persons are most subject to apoplexy between the ages of forty and sixty.

58. If the omentum protrude, it necessarily mortifies and drops off.

59. In chronic diseases of the hip-joint, if the bone protrude and return again into its socket, there is mucosity in the place.

60. In persons affected with chronic disease of the hip-joint, if the bone protrude from its socket, the limb becomes wasted and maimed, unless the part be cauterized.

SECTION VII.

1. In acute diseases, coldness of the extremities is bad.

2. Livid flesh on a diseased bone is bad.

3. Hiccup and redness of the eyes, when they supervene on vomiting, are bad.

4. A chill supervening on a sweat is not good.

5. Dysentery, or dropsy, or ecstacy coming on madness is good.

6. In a very protracted disease, loss of appetite and unmixed discharges from the bowels are bad symptoms.

7. A rigor and delirium from excessive drinking are bad.

8. From the rupture of an internal abscess, prostration of strength, vomiting, and deliquium animi result.

9. Delirium or convulsion from a flow of blood is bad.

10. Vomiting, or hiccup, or convulsion, or delirium, in ileus, is bad.

11. Pneumonia coming on pleurisy is bad.

12. Phrenitis along with pneumonia is bad.

13. Convulsion or tetanus, coming upon severe burning, is bad.

14. Stupor or delirium from a blow on the head is bad.

15. From a spitting of blood there is a spitting of pus.

16. From spitting of pus arise phthisis and a flux; and when the sputa are stopped, they die.

17. Hiccup in inflammation of the liver bad.

18. Convulsion or delirium supervening upon insomnolency is bad.

18a. Trembling upon lethargus is bad.

19. Erysipelas upon exposure of a bone (is bad?).

20. Mortification or suppuration upon erysipelas is bad.

21. Hemorrhage upon a strong pulsation in wounds is bad.

22. Suppuration upon a protracted pain of the parts about the bowels is bad.

23. Dysentery upon unmixed alvine discharges is bad.

24. Delirium upon division of the cranium, if it penetrate into the cavity of the head, is bad.

25. Convulsion upon severe purging is mortal.

26. Upon severe pain of the parts about the bowels, coldness of the extremities coming on is bad.

27. Tenesmus coming on in a case of pregnancy causes abortion.

28. Whatever piece of bone, cartilage, or nerve (tendon?) is cut off, it neither grows nor unites.

29. When strong diarrhoea supervenes in a case of leucophlegmatia, it removes the disease.

30. In those cases in which frothy discharges occur in diarrhoea there are defluxions from the head.

31. When there is a farinaceous sediment in the urine during fever, it indicates a protracted illness.

32. In those cases in which the urine is thin at first, and the sediments become bilious, an acute disease is indicated.

33. In those cases in which the urine becomes divided there is great disorder in the body.

34. When bubbles settle on the surface of the urine, they indicate disease of the kidneys, and that the complaint will be protracted.

35. When the scum on the surface is fatty and copious, it indicates acute diseases of the kidneys.

36. Whenever the aforementioned symptoms occur in nephritic diseases, and along with them acute pains about the muscles of the back, provided these be seated about the external parts, you may expect that there will be an abscess; but if the pains be rather about the internal parts, you may also rather expect that the abscess will be seated internally.

37. Haematemesis, without fever, does not prove fatal, but with fever it is bad; it is to be treated with refrigerant and styptic things.

38. Defluxions into the cavity of the chest suppurate in twenty days.

39. When a patient passes blood and clots, and is seized with strangury and pain in the perineum and pubes, disease about the bladder is indicated.

40. If the tongue suddenly lose its powers, or a part of the body become apoplectic, the affection is of a melancholic nature.

41. In hypercatharsis, of old persons, hiccup supervening is not a good symptom.

42. In a fever, is not of a bilious nature, a copious allusion of hot water upon the head removes the fever.

43. A woman does not become ambidexterous.

44. When empyema is treated either by the cautery or incision, if pure and white pus flow from the wound, the patients recover; but if mixed with blood, slimy and fetid, they die.

45. When abscess of the liver is treated by the cautery or incision, if the pus which is discharged be pure and white, the patients recover, (for in this case it is situated in the coats of the liver;) but if it resemble the lees of oil as it flows, they die.

46. Pains of the eyes are removed by drinking undiluted wine, plenteous bathing with hot water, and venesection.

47. If a dropsical patient be seized with hiccup the case is hopeless.

48. Strangury and dysuria are cured by drinking pure wine, and venesection; open the vein on the inside.

49. It is a good sign when swelling and redness on the breast seize a person very ill of quinsy, for in this case the disease is diverted outwardly.

50. When the brain is attacked with sphacelus, the patients die in three days; or if they escape these, they recover.

51. Sneezing arises from the head, owing to the brain being heated, or the cavity (ventricle) in the head being filled with humors; the air confined in it then is discharged, and makes a noise, because it comes through a narrow passage.

52. Fever supervening on painful affections of the liver removes the pain.

53. Those persons to whom it is beneficial to have blood taken from their veins, should have it done in spring.

54. In those cases where phlegm is collected between the diaphragm and the stomach, and occasions pain, as not finding a passage into either of the cavities, the disease will be carried off if the phlegm be diverted to the bladder by the veins.

55. When the liver is filled with water and bursts into the epiploon, in this case the belly is filled with water and the patient dies.

56. Anxiety, yawning, rigor,-wine drunk with an equal proportion of water, removes these complaints.

57. When tubercles (phymata) form in the urethra, if they suppurate and burst, the pain is carried off.

58. In cases of concussion of the brain produced by any cause, the patients necessarily lose their speech.

59. In a person affected with fever, when there is no swelling in the fauces, should suffocation suddenly come on, and the patient not be able to swallow, except with difficulty, it is a mortal symptom.

59a. In the case of a person oppressed by fever, if the neck be turned aside, and the patient cannot swallow, while there is no swelling in the neck, it is a mortal sign.

60. Fasting should be prescribed the those persons who have humid flesh; for fasting dries bodies.

61. When there are changes in the whole body, and the body becomes sometimes cold and sometimes hot, and the color changes, a protracted disease is indicated.

62. A copious sweat, hot or cold, constantly flowing, indicates a superabundance of humidity; we must evacuate then, in a strong person upward, and in a weak, downward.

63. Fevers, not of the intermittent type, if they become exacerbated every third day are dangerous; but if they intermit in any form whatever, this shows that they are not dangerous.

64. In cases of protracted fever, either chronic abscesses or pains in the joints come on.

65. When chronic abscesses (phymata) or pains in the joints take place after fevers, the patients are using too much food.

66. If one give to a person in fever the same food which is given to a person in good health, what is strength to the one is disease to the other.

67. We must look to the urinary evacuations, whether they resemble those of persons in health; if not at all so, they are particularly morbid, but if they are like those of healthy persons, they are not at all morbid.

68. When the dejections are allowed to stand and not shaken, and a sediment is formed like scrapings (of the bowels), in such a case it is proper to purge the bowels; and if you give ptisans before purging, the more you give the more harm you will do.

69. Crude dejections are the product of black bile; if abundant, of more copious, and if deficient, of less copious collections of it.

70. The sputa in fevers, not of an intermittent type, which are livid, streaked with blood, and fetid, are all bad, it is favorable when this evacuation, like the urinary and alvine, passes freely; and whenever any discharge is suppressed and not purged off it is bad.

71. When you wish to purge the body, you must bring it into a state favorable to evacuations; and if you wish to dispose it to evacuations upward, you must bind the belly; and if you wish to dispose it to evacuations downward, you must moisten the belly.

72. Sleep and watchfulness, both of them, when immoderate, constitute disease.

73. In fevers which do not intermit, if the external parts be cold, and the internal burning hot, and fever prevail, it is a mortal sign.

74. In a fever which does not intermit, if a lip, the nose, or an eye be distorted, if the patient lose his sense of sight or of hearing, while now in a weak state,-whatever of these symptoms occurs it is mortal.

75. Upon leucophlegmatia dropsy supervenes.

76. Upon diarrhoea dysentery.

77. Upon dysentery lientery.

78. Upon sphacelus exfoliation of the bone.

79 and 80. Upon vomiting of blood consumption, and a purging of pus upward; upon consumption a defluxion from the head; upon a defluxion diarrhoea; upon diarrhoea a stoppage of the purging upward; upon the stoppage of it death.

81. In the discharges by the bladder, the belly, and the flesh (the skin?) if the body has departed slightly from its natural condition, the disease is slight; if much, it is great; if very much, it is mortal.

82. Persons above forty years of age who are affected with frenzy, do not readily recover; the danger is less when the disease is cognate to the constitution and age.

83. In whatever diseases the eyes weep voluntarily, it is a good symptom, but when involuntarily, it is a bad.

84. When in quartan fevers blood flows from the nostrils it is a bad symptom.

85. Sweats are dangerous when they do not occur on critical days, when they are strong, and quickly forced out of the forehead, either in the form of drops or in streams, and if excessively cold and copious; for such a sweat must proceed from violence, excess of pain, and prolonged squeezing (affliction?).

86. In a chronic disease an excessive flux from the bowels is bad.

87. Those diseases which medicines do not cure, iron (the knife?) cures; those which iron cannot cure, fire cures; and those which fire cannot cure, are to be reckoned wholly incurable.

Made in the USA
Monee, IL
29 June 2021